CALM YOUR INFLAMMATION

AND RESTORE YOUR VITALITY.

8 Effective Strategies to Balance Your Immune System, Improve Gut Health, Reduce Stress, and Enhance Your Daily Well-being"

DR. ANGELINA EWELL

TABLE OF CONTENT

Introduction

In today's fast-paced world, many of us are battling chronic inflammation and its myriad effects on our health. From fatigue and digestive issues to more severe conditions like autoimmune diseases and heart problems, inflammation can be both a silent and overt disruptor of our well-being. Yet, the journey to a healthier, more vibrant life doesn't have to be complex or overwhelming.

"Calm Your Inflammation and Restore Your Vitality" offers a comprehensive guide to understanding and combating inflammation through eight effective strategies. This book is designed to empower you with the knowledge and tools necessary to balance your immune system, improve gut health, reduce stress, and enhance your daily well-being.

Understanding Inflammation and Immunity

We begin by demystifying inflammation and its crucial role in the body. While inflammation is a natural response to injury or infection, chronic inflammation can lead to a host of health problems. By understanding the science behind inflammation and the immune system's function, you can better grasp the importance of managing inflammation for overall health.

Nourishing Your Body: Anti-Inflammatory Nutrition

What we eat plays a significant role in either fueling or fighting inflammation. This section delves into the best foods to include in your diet, how to create balanced, anti-inflammatory meals, and the supplements that can support immune health. Learn how to make nutrition work for you in the fight against inflammation.

Gut Health: The Foundation of Wellness

Your gut is at the center of your health. A healthy gut not only aids digestion but also supports immune function and reduces inflammation. Explore the gut-inflammation connection and discover practical strategies for improving and maintaining gut health through diet and lifestyle changes.

Stress Reduction Techniques

Chronic stress is a major contributor to inflammation. This chapter provides a range of stress reduction techniques, including mindfulness, meditation, and other effective strategies to help you manage stress and reduce its impact on your body.

The Power of Physical Activity

Regular physical activity is crucial for reducing inflammation and boosting immune function. Learn about the best types of exercise for combating inflammation and how to develop a consistent and enjoyable exercise routine.

Restorative Sleep for Vitality

Quality sleep is essential for controlling inflammation and maintaining overall health. This section offers tips for improving sleep quality, creating a sleep-friendly environment, and understanding the role of sleep in managing inflammation.

Detoxifying Your Life

Reducing your exposure to environmental toxins can significantly impact inflammation levels. Discover natural detox methods, how to reduce toxin exposure, and ways to support your body's natural detoxification processes.

Building a Sustainable Lifestyle

Integrating these strategies into your daily life is key to long-term health and vitality. This final chapter provides guidance on how to make lasting changes, track your progress, and stay motivated on your journey to a healthier, inflammation-free life.

By following these eight effective strategies, you can take control of your health, calm your inflammation, and restore your vitality. This book is your roadmap to a balanced immune system, improved gut health, reduced stress, and enhanced daily well-being. Start your journey today and unlock the vibrant life you deserve.

Chapter 1

Understanding Inflammation and Immunity

Inflammation is a complex biological response that plays a critical role in the body's defense mechanisms. It is essential for healing and protection against infection, yet when unregulated, it can become a source of chronic disease and discomfort. To effectively manage and mitigate inflammation, it is crucial to understand its underlying science and its relationship with the immune system.

The Science of Inflammation

Inflammation is the body's natural response to injury, infection, or harmful stimuli. It is a vital part of the immune system's protective mechanism. The process involves a series of coordinated steps:

1. **Recognition of Harm:** When the body detects a pathogen, damaged cells, or irritants, immune cells recognize these threats and initiate the inflammatory response.
2. **Recruitment of Immune Cells:** Signals such as cytokines and chemokines are released, attracting white blood cells to the affected area.
3. **Elimination of the Threat:** White blood cells, including neutrophils and macrophages, work to eliminate the pathogens or damaged cells.

4. **Resolution and Healing**: Once the threat is neutralized, anti-inflammatory signals are released to cease the inflammatory response, allowing tissue repair and healing.

This process is vital for survival, as it helps to contain and eradicate infections and facilitate tissue repair. However, when inflammation persists or is improperly regulated, it can lead to chronic inflammation, contributing to various diseases such as arthritis, cardiovascular disease, and even cancer.

How Your Immune System Works

The immune system is a complex network of cells, tissues, and organs that work together to defend the body against harmful invaders. It consists of two main components: the innate immune system and the adaptive immune system.

1. **Innate Immune System:** This is the body's first line of defense. It includes physical barriers like the skin and mucous membranes, as well as immune cells such as macrophages and neutrophils that respond quickly to a wide range of pathogens in a non-specific manner.

2. **Adaptive Immune System:** This system provides a more targeted and long-lasting response. It involves lymphocytes (B cells and T cells) that recognize specific antigens and

create memory cells for faster responses upon future exposures to the same pathogen.

Both systems work in harmony to protect the body. The innate immune response triggers inflammation to rapidly deal with threats, while the adaptive immune response takes longer to activate but provides a more precise and long-term defense.

Chronic vs. Acute Inflammation

Understanding the difference between acute and chronic inflammation is crucial for recognizing their impacts on health:

1. **Acute Inflammation:** This is a short-term response to injury or infection, characterized by redness, heat, swelling, and pain. It is a beneficial and necessary process that typically resolves once the body has dealt with the threat. Examples include the inflammation you experience with a cut, sprain, or infection like the flu.

2. **Chronic Inflammation:** When inflammation persists over a long period, it becomes chronic. This can occur due to unresolved infections, ongoing exposure to irritants, autoimmune reactions, or metabolic imbalances. Chronic inflammation is often subtle and less noticeable than acute inflammation, but it can cause significant damage over

time, contributing to diseases such as diabetes, heart disease, and autoimmune disorders.

Chronic inflammation is particularly insidious because it can silently damage tissues and organs without obvious symptoms. Managing chronic inflammation requires a holistic approach, addressing diet, lifestyle, and underlying health conditions to restore balance and health.

Understanding the science of inflammation and the workings of the immune system is fundamental to managing health and well-being. By recognizing the difference between acute and chronic inflammation, and knowing how to support your immune system, you can take proactive steps to reduce inflammation, enhance your vitality, and prevent chronic diseases. This knowledge serves as the foundation for the effective strategies presented in this book, guiding you towards a healthier, inflammation-free life.

Chapter 2

Nourishing Your Body: Anti-Inflammatory Nutrition

Diet plays a crucial role in managing inflammation and maintaining overall health. The right foods can help reduce inflammation, support immune function, and promote vitality. This chapter explores foods that fight inflammation, how to create balanced, anti-inflammatory meals, and the essential supplements that can enhance your immune health.

Foods That Fight Inflammation

Certain foods are known for their anti-inflammatory properties, helping to reduce chronic inflammation and support overall health. Incorporating these foods into your diet can significantly impact your well-being:

1. **Fruits and Vegetables**: Rich in antioxidants and phytonutrients, fruits and vegetables help combat oxidative stress and inflammation. Berries (such as blueberries, strawberries, and raspberries), leafy greens (like spinach and kale), and cruciferous vegetables (such as broccoli and Brussels sprouts) are particularly effective.

2. **Healthy Fats:** Omega-3 fatty acids found in fatty fish (like salmon, mackerel, and sardines), flaxseeds, chia seeds, and walnuts are potent anti-inflammatory agents. Extra virgin olive oil, rich in monounsaturated fats, also has anti-inflammatory benefits.

3. **Whole Grains:** Whole grains like brown rice, quinoa, and oats provide fiber and essential nutrients that help regulate the body's inflammatory response. Choose whole grains over refined grains to maximize their benefits.

4. **Nuts and Seeds:** Almonds, walnuts, flaxseeds, chia seeds, and sunflower seeds are packed with healthy fats, protein, and antioxidants that help reduce inflammation.

5. **Herbs and Spices:** Turmeric, ginger, garlic, and cinnamon are known for their anti-inflammatory properties. Incorporating these herbs and spices into your meals can enhance flavor and reduce inflammation.

6. **Green Tea:** Rich in polyphenols and antioxidants, green tea has been shown to reduce inflammation and support overall health.

Creating Balanced, Anti-Inflammatory Meals

To maximize the benefits of anti-inflammatory foods, it's important to create balanced meals that provide all the necessary nutrients your body needs. Here are some tips for designing anti-inflammatory meals:

1. **Focus on Whole Foods:** Prioritize whole, unprocessed foods. Avoid processed foods, refined sugars, and unhealthy fats that can increase inflammation.

2. **Include a Variety of Colors:** Aim to fill your plate with a variety of colorful fruits and vegetables. Each color represents different phytonutrients that contribute to reducing inflammation and supporting health.

3. **Balance Macronutrients:** Ensure each meal contains a balance of protein, healthy fats, and complex carbohydrates. This helps maintain stable blood sugar levels and reduces inflammation.

4. **Incorporate Anti-Inflammatory Ingredients:** Use herbs, spices, and healthy fats liberally in your cooking. Experiment with recipes that include turmeric, ginger, garlic, and extra virgin olive oil.

5. **Hydrate Well:** Drink plenty of water throughout the day. Proper hydration is essential for maintaining healthy bodily functions and reducing inflammation.

Essential Supplements for Immune Health

In addition to a balanced diet, certain supplements can support your immune system and help reduce inflammation. Here are some essential supplements to consider:

1. **Omega-3 Fatty Acids:** If you don't consume enough fatty fish, consider an omega-3 supplement. Fish oil or algae oil supplements can provide the necessary EPA and DHA to reduce inflammation.

2. **Vitamin D:** Vitamin D is crucial for immune function and has anti-inflammatory properties. Many people are deficient in vitamin D, so supplementation may be necessary, especially during the winter months.

3. **Probiotics:** A healthy gut microbiome is essential for controlling inflammation. Probiotic supplements can help balance gut bacteria and support overall gut health.

4. **Curcumin:** The active compound in turmeric, curcumin, has powerful anti-inflammatory effects. Taking a curcumin supplement can enhance its bioavailability and provide significant benefits.

5. **Vitamin C:** Known for its immune-boosting properties, vitamin C also helps reduce inflammation. It can be particularly beneficial during times of stress or illness.

6. **Magnesium:** This essential mineral helps regulate inflammation and supports numerous bodily functions. Many people have inadequate magnesium levels, so supplementation can be beneficial.

Nourishing your body with anti-inflammatory foods, creating balanced meals, and incorporating essential supplements are key steps in managing inflammation and supporting overall health. By making these dietary adjustments, you can reduce chronic inflammation, boost your immune system, and enhance your vitality. This approach to nutrition is a foundational element of the comprehensive strategies outlined in this book, guiding you toward a healthier, inflammation-free life.

Chapter 3

Gut Health: The Foundation of Wellness

The health of your gut plays a fundamental role in overall wellness. An optimally functioning gut not only aids in digestion but also supports immune function, regulates inflammation, and impacts mental health. Understanding the gut-inflammation connection, the role of probiotics and prebiotics, and effective strategies for gut health is essential for maintaining a balanced and healthy body.

The Gut-Inflammation Connection

The gut, or gastrointestinal tract, is often referred to as the "second brain" due to its significant influence on overall health. A healthy gut supports a balanced immune response and helps regulate inflammation throughout the body. Here's how the gut and inflammation are interconnected:

1. **Gut Barrier Function:** The gut lining acts as a barrier between the internal environment and the external world. When this barrier is compromised, a condition known as "leaky gut" can occur, allowing harmful substances to enter the bloodstream and trigger an inflammatory response.

2. **Gut Microbiome:** The gut microbiome, a diverse community of microorganisms residing in the digestive tract, plays a crucial role in modulating inflammation. A healthy, balanced microbiome helps maintain gut barrier integrity and supports immune function. Imbalances in gut bacteria can lead to chronic inflammation and contribute to various health issues.

3. **Immune System Interaction:** The gut-associated lymphoid tissue (GALT) is a critical component of the immune system located in the gut. It monitors and responds to pathogens and other antigens. A well-functioning GALT helps prevent excessive inflammation by maintaining immune tolerance and promoting a balanced immune response.

Probiotics, Prebiotics, and Gut-Friendly Foods

Supporting gut health involves incorporating specific foods and supplements that foster a healthy microbiome and support digestive function:

1. **Probiotics:** Probiotics are live beneficial bacteria that help restore and maintain a healthy gut microbiome. Common sources include fermented foods like yogurt, kefir, sauerkraut, kimchi, and miso. Probiotic supplements can

also provide targeted strains that may be beneficial for specific health concerns.

2. **Prebiotics:** Prebiotics are non-digestible fibers that serve as food for beneficial gut bacteria. They help stimulate the growth and activity of probiotics. Foods rich in prebiotics include garlic, onions, leeks, bananas, asparagus, and chicory root.

3. **Gut-Friendly Foods:** Incorporate foods that support gut health and reduce inflammation. These include:

- **Fiber-Rich Foods:** Whole grains, fruits, and vegetables provide essential fiber that supports digestive health and nourishes beneficial gut bacteria.

- **Bone Broth:** Rich in collagen and amino acids, bone broth helps heal and maintain the gut lining.

- **Healthy Fats:** Omega-3 fatty acids from sources like fatty fish, flaxseeds, and chia seeds support anti-inflammatory processes in the gut.

- **Anti-Inflammatory Spices:** Turmeric and ginger have been shown to reduce gut inflammation and support overall digestive health.

Strategies for Healing and Maintaining Gut Health

To promote and sustain optimal gut health, consider the following strategies:

1. **Adopt a Balanced Diet:** Focus on a diet rich in whole, unprocessed foods, including a variety of fruits, vegetables, whole grains, lean proteins, and healthy fats. Avoid excessive consumption of processed foods, refined sugars, and artificial additives that can negatively impact gut health.

2. **Stay Hydrated:** Adequate hydration is essential for digestive health. Drinking plenty of water helps maintain the mucosal lining of the intestines and supports overall digestive function.

3. **Manage Stress:** Chronic stress can disrupt gut function and contribute to inflammation. Incorporate stress-reducing practices such as mindfulness, meditation, yoga, and regular physical activity to support gut health.

4. **Exercise Regularly:** Physical activity promotes a healthy gut microbiome and supports overall digestive function. Aim for at least 150 minutes of moderate-intensity exercise per week.

5. **Prioritize Sleep:** Quality sleep is essential for maintaining gut health. Aim for 7-9 hours of restful sleep per night to support overall wellness and gut function.

6. **Avoid Overuse of Antibiotics:** Antibiotics can disrupt the balance of gut bacteria. Use them only when prescribed by a healthcare professional and consider taking probiotics to help restore gut flora afterward.

7. **Monitor Food Sensitivities:** Identifying and avoiding foods that trigger digestive issues can help prevent inflammation and support gut health. Common culprits include gluten, dairy, and certain high-FODMAP foods.

Gut health is a cornerstone of overall well-being, influencing inflammation, immune function, and digestive health. By understanding the gut-inflammation connection, incorporating probiotics and prebiotics, and adopting effective strategies for gut care, you can support a healthy microbiome, reduce inflammation, and enhance your overall vitality. This holistic approach to gut health is integral to the comprehensive strategies presented in this book, guiding you toward a healthier, more balanced life.

Chapter 4

Stress Reduction Techniques

Stress is a powerful force that can significantly impact your health and well-being. Chronic stress, in particular, can exacerbate inflammation, compromise immune function, and lead to a range of physical and emotional issues. Understanding the relationship between stress and inflammation, and employing effective stress reduction techniques, can help restore balance and improve overall health.

The Impact of Stress on Inflammation

Stress triggers a cascade of physiological responses that can contribute to chronic inflammation:

1. **Stress Hormones:** When you experience stress, your body releases stress hormones such as cortisol and adrenaline. While these hormones are beneficial in the short term for dealing with immediate threats, prolonged elevated levels can lead to increased inflammation and other health issues.

2. **Immune System Disruption:** Chronic stress can alter immune function, leading to an overactive or dysregulated immune response. This imbalance can contribute to

persistent inflammation and increase susceptibility to inflammatory diseases.

3. **Gut Health:** Stress can negatively affect gut health, leading to a condition known as "leaky gut," where the gut lining becomes compromised. This allows toxins and inflammatory agents to enter the bloodstream, further exacerbating inflammation.

4. **Behavioral Factors:** Stress often leads to unhealthy coping mechanisms such as poor diet choices, lack of exercise, and disrupted sleep. These factors can collectively contribute to increased inflammation and deteriorate overall health.

Mindfulness and Meditation Practices

Mindfulness and meditation are powerful techniques for reducing stress and mitigating its effects on the body. These practices can help calm the mind, lower stress hormone levels, and promote a state of relaxation and well-being:

1. **Mindfulness:** Mindfulness involves paying attention to the present moment with openness and non-judgment. It can help you become more aware of stress triggers and develop a more balanced perspective. Techniques include mindful breathing, mindful eating, and body scan meditations.

2. **Meditation:** Meditation practices, such as guided meditation, loving-kindness meditation, and transcendental

meditation, can help reduce stress and promote relaxation. Regular meditation practice has been shown to lower cortisol levels, improve emotional regulation, and enhance overall mental health.

3. **Deep Breathing Exercises:** Deep breathing exercises, such as diaphragmatic breathing or box breathing, help activate the parasympathetic nervous system, which counteracts the stress response and induces a state of calm.

4. **Progressive Muscle Relaxation:** This technique involves systematically tensing and then relaxing different muscle groups in the body. It helps release physical tension associated with stress and promotes relaxation.

Effective Stress Management Strategies

In addition to mindfulness and meditation, various strategies can help manage and reduce stress effectively:

1. **Establish a Routine:** Creating a consistent daily routine can provide structure and predictability, reducing feelings of chaos and stress. Incorporate regular sleep, balanced meals, and scheduled breaks into your routine.

2. **Physical Activity:** Regular exercise is a powerful stress reliever. Activities like walking, jogging, yoga, and strength training release endorphins, which improve mood

and reduce stress. Aim for at least 150 minutes of moderate-intensity exercise per week.

3. **Healthy Diet:** Eating a balanced diet with plenty of fruits, vegetables, whole grains, lean proteins, and healthy fats supports overall health and helps manage stress. Avoid excessive caffeine, sugar, and processed foods, which can exacerbate stress.

4. **Social Support:** Connecting with friends, family, or support groups can provide emotional support and reduce feelings of isolation. Sharing your experiences and seeking advice can help you cope with stress more effectively.

5. **Time Management:** Effective time management techniques, such as setting priorities, breaking tasks into manageable steps, and avoiding procrastination, can reduce stress related to workload and deadlines.

6. **Hobbies and Relaxation:** Engage in activities that you enjoy and that help you relax. Whether it's reading, gardening, painting, or listening to music, taking time for hobbies can provide a much-needed break from stress.

7. **Professional Help:** If stress becomes overwhelming or persistent, consider seeking help from a mental health professional. Therapy, counseling, and other forms of professional support can provide valuable tools and strategies for managing stress.

Managing stress is crucial for reducing inflammation, maintaining a healthy immune system, and enhancing overall well-being. By understanding the impact of stress on inflammation and incorporating mindfulness, meditation, and effective stress management strategies into your daily life, you can promote relaxation, improve health, and restore balance. These techniques form an integral part of the holistic approach to health outlined in this book, guiding you toward a more resilient and vibrant life.

Chapter 5

The Power of Physical Activity

Physical activity is a cornerstone of a healthy lifestyle, offering a multitude of benefits that extend beyond weight management and cardiovascular health. One of the most profound impacts of regular exercise is its ability to reduce inflammation and bolster immune function. Understanding how exercise influences these aspects of health, the most effective types of exercise for reducing inflammation, and how to develop a consistent routine can significantly enhance your well-being.

Benefits of Exercise for Inflammation and Immunity

Engaging in regular physical activity has a range of benefits for both inflammation and immune system function:

1. **Reduction in Inflammation:** Exercise has been shown to lower levels of systemic inflammation. It helps decrease the production of pro-inflammatory cytokines and increases the release of anti-inflammatory cytokines. This shift reduces overall inflammation and helps prevent chronic diseases associated with inflammation.

2. **Improved Immune Function:** Regular exercise enhances the efficiency of the immune system. It stimulates the

production of immune cells, improves circulation, and helps the body more effectively respond to infections. Exercise also supports the production of antibodies and improves the function of immune cells like T cells and macrophages.

3. **Enhanced Mood and Stress Management:** Physical activity promotes the release of endorphins, which improve mood and help manage stress. Reducing stress and improving mental health can indirectly support immune function and reduce inflammation.

4. **Better Sleep Quality:** Regular exercise contributes to improved sleep quality and duration. Quality sleep is crucial for immune health and helps regulate inflammation by allowing the body to repair and recover.

Best Exercises for Reducing Inflammation

Certain types of exercise are particularly effective in managing inflammation and supporting overall health:

1. **Aerobic Exercise:** Activities such as walking, jogging, swimming, and cycling are excellent for reducing inflammation. Aerobic exercise improves cardiovascular health, enhances circulation, and helps regulate inflammatory markers. Aim for at least 150 minutes of moderate-intensity aerobic exercise per week.

2. **Strength Training:** Resistance exercises, such as weightlifting, bodyweight exercises, and resistance band workouts, are beneficial for reducing inflammation and building muscle mass. Strength training helps improve metabolic health and supports joint function, which can mitigate inflammatory responses.

3. **Yoga and Stretching:** Yoga and stretching exercises promote flexibility, reduce muscle tension, and improve relaxation. These practices also enhance mind-body connection, helping to manage stress and inflammation. Incorporate yoga sessions or stretching routines into your weekly exercise regimen.

4. **Low-Impact Activities:** Activities such as Tai Chi and Pilates offer low-impact exercise options that are gentle on the joints while still providing significant benefits for inflammation and overall health. These exercises improve balance, coordination, and muscle strength.

5. **High-Intensity Interval Training (HIIT):** HIIT involves alternating between short bursts of intense exercise and periods of lower-intensity recovery. This type of workout has been shown to improve cardiovascular fitness, reduce inflammation, and enhance metabolic function. Incorporate HIIT sessions 1-2 times per week for optimal results.

Developing a Consistent Exercise Routine

Establishing a regular exercise routine is key to reaping the benefits of physical activity for inflammation and immune health. Here are some strategies to help you build and maintain a consistent exercise routine:

1. **Set Clear Goals:** Define specific, achievable goals for your fitness routine. Whether it's improving endurance, building strength, or increasing flexibility, having clear objectives will help keep you motivated.

2. **Create a Schedule:** Designate specific days and times for exercise in your weekly schedule. Treat these sessions as important appointments to ensure consistency.

3. **Choose Activities You Enjoy:** Select exercises that you find enjoyable and engaging. Enjoyable activities are more likely to become a regular part of your routine.

4. **Start Slowly and Progress Gradually:** If you're new to exercise or returning after a break, start with moderate-intensity activities and gradually increase the intensity and duration as your fitness level improves.

5. **Mix It Up:** Incorporate a variety of exercises into your routine to prevent boredom and target different aspects of fitness. Combining aerobic exercise, strength training,

flexibility work, and low-impact activities provides comprehensive benefits.

6. **Track Your Progress:** Keep a record of your workouts, including duration, intensity, and any improvements you notice. Tracking progress helps you stay motivated and see the benefits of your efforts.

7. **Listen to Your Body:** Pay attention to how your body responds to exercise. Rest and recovery are essential components of a balanced routine, so allow time for rest and avoid overtraining.

8. **Seek Professional Guidance:** If you're unsure how to start or design an exercise routine, consider consulting a fitness professional or personal trainer. They can provide personalized guidance and help you develop a safe and effective plan.

Physical activity is a powerful tool for reducing inflammation, enhancing immune function, and supporting overall health. By incorporating a variety of exercises into your routine and developing a consistent approach to physical activity, you can reap the significant benefits of improved inflammation control and immune health. Embracing regular exercise as a fundamental part of your lifestyle is essential for achieving long-term well-being and vitality.

Chapter 6

Restorative Sleep for Vitality

Restorative sleep is a vital component of overall health and well-being. Quality sleep supports various physiological processes, including immune function and inflammation regulation. Understanding how sleep impacts inflammation, employing strategies to improve sleep quality, and creating a sleep-friendly environment can significantly enhance vitality and overall health.

Understanding the Role of Sleep in Inflammation

Sleep plays a crucial role in managing inflammation and supporting immune function. The relationship between sleep and inflammation is complex but essential for maintaining health:

1. **Regulation of Inflammatory Markers:** Adequate sleep helps regulate the production of inflammatory cytokines and other markers. Poor sleep or sleep deprivation can lead to increased levels of pro-inflammatory cytokines, contributing to chronic inflammation and associated health issues.

2. **Immune System Function:** During sleep, the body produces and releases cytokines that help fight infections and inflammation. Quality sleep supports the immune

system's ability to respond to pathogens and repair damaged tissues.

3. **Hormonal Balance:** Sleep affects the balance of hormones such as cortisol, which plays a role in the body's stress response and inflammation. Disrupted sleep can lead to hormonal imbalances that exacerbate inflammation.

4. **Restoration and Recovery:** Sleep is a time for the body to repair and regenerate. It allows for cellular repair, muscle recovery, and the restoration of various bodily functions that help control inflammation and support overall health.

Tips for Improving Sleep Quality

Enhancing sleep quality involves adopting habits and practices that promote restful and restorative sleep. Here are some effective strategies:

1. **Maintain a Consistent Sleep Schedule:** Go to bed and wake up at the same time every day, even on weekends. Consistency helps regulate your internal clock and improve the quality of your sleep.

2. **Create a Relaxing Bedtime Routine:** Establish a calming pre-sleep routine to signal your body that it's time to wind down. Activities such as reading, gentle stretching, or practicing relaxation techniques can help prepare your body for sleep.

3. **Limit Exposure to Screens:** Avoid screens (phones, tablets, computers, TVs) at least an hour before bedtime. The blue light emitted by screens can interfere with melatonin production, making it harder to fall asleep.

4. **Avoid Stimulants and Heavy Meals:** Refrain from consuming caffeine, nicotine, and heavy or large meals close to bedtime. These substances can disrupt sleep and make it more difficult to fall and stay asleep.

5. **Stay Active During the Day:** Regular physical activity can promote better sleep. Aim for at least 30 minutes of moderate exercise most days, but avoid vigorous activity too close to bedtime, as it may interfere with sleep

6. **Manage Stress and Anxiety:** Practice stress-reducing techniques such as mindfulness, meditation, or deep breathing exercises to calm your mind and prepare for restful sleep.

7. **Monitor Sleep Environment:** Ensure your sleep environment is conducive to rest. Maintain a cool, dark, and quiet room, and invest in a comfortable mattress and pillows.

Creating a Sleep-Friendly Environment

The environment in which you sleep plays a significant role in sleep quality. Here are key considerations for creating a sleep-friendly environment:

1. **Optimize Room Temperature:** Keep your bedroom at a cool, comfortable temperature. The ideal range for most people is between 60-67°F (15-19°C). A cool room helps promote deeper, more restorative sleep.

2. **Minimize Light Exposure:** Darkness signals your body that it's time to sleep. Use blackout curtains or an eye mask to block external light. Dim the lights in your bedroom in the hour leading up to bedtime.

3. **Reduce Noise Levels:** Create a quiet sleeping environment by using earplugs, white noise machines, or fans to mask disruptive sounds. Consistent background noise can help promote better sleep.

4. **Invest in Quality Bedding:** Choose a comfortable mattress and pillows that support proper alignment and comfort. The right bedding can enhance sleep quality and prevent discomfort during the night.

5. **Keep Electronics Out of the Bedroom:** Designate your bedroom as a space for sleep and relaxation. Avoid

bringing work, screens, or other distractions into the bedroom to create a more restful environment.

6. **Maintain Cleanliness and Organization:** A tidy and clean bedroom can contribute to a more relaxing atmosphere. Keep your sleep environment free of clutter and ensure bedding is fresh and comfortable.

Restorative sleep is essential for managing inflammation, supporting immune function, and enhancing overall vitality. By understanding the critical role of sleep in health, implementing strategies to improve sleep quality, and creating a sleep-friendly environment, you can promote better rest and achieve a higher level of well-being. Prioritizing sleep as a fundamental aspect of your health routine will help you maintain balance and support your body's natural healing processes.

Chapter 7

Detoxifying Your Life

Detoxifying your life involves adopting practices that help reduce the burden of toxins on your body and support its natural detoxification processes. By incorporating natural detox methods, minimizing exposure to environmental toxins, and enhancing your body's detoxification systems, you can improve overall health and vitality. Here's how to effectively detoxify your life:

Natural Detox Methods

Natural detox methods focus on promoting the body's innate ability to cleanse and rejuvenate itself. These methods are gentle and support overall health without extreme or restrictive measures:

1. **Hydration:** Drinking plenty of water is fundamental to the detoxification process. Water helps flush out toxins through the kidneys and supports overall bodily functions. Aim for at least 8 glasses of water per day, and consider adding herbal teas like dandelion or ginger, which have natural detoxifying properties.

2. **Nutrient-Rich Diet:** A diet rich in fruits, vegetables, whole grains, and lean proteins supports the body's detoxification systems. Foods such as leafy greens, berries, citrus fruits,

garlic, and cruciferous vegetables (e.g., broccoli, Brussels sprouts) contain antioxidants and nutrients that aid in detoxification.

3. **Juicing and Smoothies:** Incorporating fresh vegetable and fruit juices or smoothies into your diet can provide a concentrated dose of nutrients and antioxidants. Green juices made from kale, spinach, cucumber, and lemon are particularly beneficial for supporting detoxification.

4. **Herbal Supplements:** Certain herbs and supplements can aid in detoxification. Milk thistle, for example, is known for its liver-supporting properties, while turmeric has anti-inflammatory and antioxidant benefits. Consult with a healthcare provider before adding new supplements to your routine.

5. **Regular Exercise:** Physical activity promotes circulation and sweating, both of which help expel toxins from the body. Incorporate activities like walking, running, yoga, or strength training into your routine to support the detoxification process.

6. **Sauna Therapy:** Using a sauna can help induce sweating, which aids in the elimination of toxins through the skin. Regular sauna sessions can support the detoxification process and promote relaxation.

Reducing Exposure to Toxins

Minimizing exposure to environmental and dietary toxins is crucial for supporting overall health and reducing the toxic load on the body:

1. **Choose Organic Foods:** Opt for organic produce and products when possible to reduce exposure to pesticides, herbicides, and other chemicals. Washing fruits and vegetables thoroughly can also help remove residues.

2. **Avoid Processed Foods:** Processed and packaged foods often contain artificial additives, preservatives, and high levels of sugar and sodium. Focus on whole, unprocessed foods to minimize intake of harmful substances.

3. **Reduce Exposure to Environmental Pollutants:** Limit exposure to environmental pollutants by using air purifiers, avoiding smoking, and minimizing time spent in heavily polluted areas. Ensure proper ventilation in your home to reduce indoor air pollution.

4. **Be Mindful of Personal Care Products:** Many personal care and household products contain chemicals that can be absorbed through the skin or inhaled. Choose natural or organic products for skincare, cleaning, and personal hygiene.

5. **Avoid Heavy Metals:** Minimize exposure to heavy metals by choosing safe sources of water, avoiding fish high in mercury, and using stainless steel or glass containers instead of plastic.

6. **Filter Drinking Water:** Use a high-quality water filter to remove contaminants and toxins from your drinking water. Regularly replace filters according to manufacturer guidelines to ensure effectiveness.

Supporting Your Body's Natural Detox Processes

The body has built-in systems for detoxification, including the liver, kidneys, and lymphatic system. Supporting these natural processes can enhance their effectiveness and overall health:

1. **Support Liver Health:** The liver plays a central role in detoxification. Support liver function by consuming liver-friendly foods such as beets, leafy greens, and artichokes. Avoid excessive alcohol consumption and other liver stressors.

2. **Enhance Kidney Function:** The kidneys filter toxins from the blood and excrete them in urine. Support kidney health by staying hydrated and consuming foods that promote kidney function, such as cranberries, apples, and watermelon.

3. **Promote Lymphatic Health:** The lymphatic system helps remove waste products from the body. Support lymphatic function through regular exercise, dry brushing, and consuming foods that promote lymphatic health, such as garlic and ginger.

4. **Practice Stress Management:** Chronic stress can impair the body's ability to detoxify and recover. Engage in stress-reducing practices such as mindfulness, meditation, and deep breathing to support overall well-being.

5. **Ensure Adequate Sleep:** Quality sleep is essential for the body's detoxification processes. Aim for 7-9 hours of restful sleep per night to support optimal liver function and overall health.

6. **Regular Detox Practices:** Incorporate regular detox practices such as intermittent fasting or periodic detox diets under professional guidance. These practices can support the body's natural detoxification processes and enhance overall health.

Detoxifying your life involves a multifaceted approach that includes natural detox methods, reducing exposure to toxins, and supporting your body's innate detoxification systems. By adopting these strategies, you can improve health, enhance vitality, and create a more balanced and toxin-free lifestyle. Prioritizing these practices will contribute to overall well-being and help your body function at its best.

Chapter 8

Building a Sustainable Lifestyle

Creating a sustainable lifestyle involves integrating practices that support long-term health, balance, and well-being. By incorporating anti-inflammatory strategies into daily life, developing long-term health and vitality strategies, and tracking progress to maintain motivation, you can build a lifestyle that promotes lasting wellness and vitality. Here's how to effectively build and sustain a healthy lifestyle:

Integrating Anti-Inflammatory Practices into Daily Life

Adopting anti-inflammatory practices consistently is key to maintaining long-term health and preventing chronic diseases. Here are practical ways to incorporate these practices into your daily routine:

1. **Adopt a Balanced Diet:** Incorporate anti-inflammatory foods into your meals, such as leafy greens, berries, nuts, seeds, fatty fish, and whole grains. Use herbs and spices like turmeric, ginger, and garlic in your cooking for their anti-inflammatory properties. Aim to fill half your plate with vegetables and fruits at every meal.

2. **Prioritize Regular Physical Activity:** Engage in a variety of exercises, including aerobic activities, strength training, and flexibility exercises. Aim for at least 150 minutes of moderate-intensity aerobic exercise per week, along with strength training exercises twice a week. Incorporate activities like walking, yoga, or swimming that you enjoy to maintain consistency.

3. **Practice Mindfulness and Stress Management:** Integrate mindfulness practices such as meditation, deep breathing exercises, or yoga into your daily routine. Schedule regular time for relaxation and stress-reducing activities to manage stress effectively.

4. **Ensure Quality Sleep:** Establish a consistent sleep schedule and create a sleep-friendly environment. Prioritize 7-9 hours of restful sleep each night to support your body's recovery and detoxification processes.

5. **Stay Hydrated:** Drink plenty of water throughout the day to support bodily functions and aid in detoxification. Consider incorporating herbal teas that have anti-inflammatory benefits, such as chamomile or green tea.

6. **Reduce Toxin Exposure:** Make conscious choices to reduce exposure to environmental toxins. Opt for natural cleaning products, personal care items, and foods free from artificial additives and chemicals.

Long-Term Strategies for Health and Vitality

Building and maintaining a sustainable lifestyle requires long-term commitment and strategic planning. Consider these strategies to support ongoing health and vitality:

1. **Set Realistic Goals:** Establish clear, achievable health goals that align with your lifestyle. Break down larger goals into smaller, manageable steps, and set deadlines to track your progress.

2. **Create a Routine:** Develop a daily or weekly routine that incorporates healthy habits. Consistent routines help make healthy practices a natural part of your lifestyle, reducing the effort required to maintain them.

3. **Focus on Balanced Nutrition:** Plan and prepare balanced meals that include a variety of nutrient-dense foods. Meal prepping and making healthy food choices in advance can help you stay on track with your nutrition goals.

4. **Engage in Continuous Learning:** Stay informed about the latest health and wellness research. Educate yourself on new strategies, techniques, and trends that can enhance your lifestyle and address any health concerns.

5. **Build a Support System:** Surround yourself with supportive individuals who share similar health goals. Join wellness groups, connect with a health coach, or engage

with friends and family to create a network that encourages and motivates you.

6. **Incorporate Rest and Recovery:** Ensure that your routine includes adequate time for rest and recovery. Balance periods of activity with relaxation to prevent burnout and support overall well-being.

7. **Adapt and Evolve:** Be open to adjusting your strategies as needed. Life circumstances and health needs may change, so flexibility in your approach allows you to adapt and maintain a sustainable lifestyle.

Tracking Progress and Staying Motivated

Monitoring your progress and maintaining motivation are crucial for sustaining a healthy lifestyle. Here are effective strategies to keep yourself on track:

1. **Keep a Journal:** Maintain a health journal to record your daily activities, food intake, exercise routines, and any changes in your well-being. Regularly review your entries to identify patterns, celebrate achievements, and make adjustments as needed.

2. **Use Technology:** Leverage apps and tools that track your fitness, nutrition, and overall health. Many apps offer features to monitor progress, set goals, and provide reminders to stay on track.

3. **Set Milestones:** Establish short-term and long-term milestones to measure your progress. Celebrating small victories and reaching milestones provides motivation and reinforces your commitment to a sustainable lifestyle.

4. **Regular Self-Assessment:** Periodically assess your health and wellness goals. Evaluate what's working well and identify areas for improvement. Adjust your strategies based on your self-assessment to stay aligned with your objectives.

5. **Reward Yourself:** Set up a reward system for achieving your goals. Choose rewards that are meaningful and aligned with your health goals, such as a relaxing massage, a new workout outfit, or a fun activity.

6. **Seek Professional Support:** Consider working with health professionals, such as a nutritionist, personal trainer, or therapist, to provide guidance, support, and accountability. Professional advice can help you navigate challenges and maintain progress.

Building a sustainable lifestyle involves integrating anti-inflammatory practices into daily life, developing long-term strategies for health and vitality, and effectively tracking progress and staying motivated. By incorporating these elements into your routine, you can create a lifestyle that supports enduring well-being, enhances vitality, and promotes a balanced and healthy life.

Consistency, adaptability, and commitment are key to achieving and maintaining your health goals.